Quick and Simple Strength Training Workouts for Seniors Over 60

At-Home Workouts for Seniors 60+ to Improve Strength, Flexibility and Posture with 20-Minute Power-Packed Exercises

[BONUS: AUDIOBOOK + VIDEO COURSES]

Carol Bolden

Copyright © 2024 by Carol Bolden

Printed in USA

First Edition: Feb, 2024

Here is one of the biggest bonuses I promised you…

A full Audiobook on the **Quick and Simple Strength Training Workouts for Seniors Over 60**

To get access to it, kindly type in this link on your browser:

https://drive.google.com/file/d/1V4L0FYiKUt3mYHV6K7Qxt690po4Ot aKv/view?usp=sharing

OR

Scan the below QR code to gain access.

GET THE COMPLETE VIDEO COURSES AT THE END OF THIS BOOK

Table Of Content

Introduction

Quick and Easy Strength Training Workouts for elders Over 60 seeks to dispel the myth that getting older is a barrier to fitness and motivate a new generation of active, robust, and healthy elders. This book provides a thorough overview of at-home exercises intended especially for those 60 years of age and over. It is filled with useful tips and information that may help seniors become more flexible, strong, and aware of their posture. Seniors may reap a number of advantages from enhanced energy and mobility to a lower chance of injury and chronic disease by simply adding a few 20-minute, high-intensity activities to their daily routines.

Because of their knowledge, wisdom, and experience, seniors have always been regarded and esteemed in civilizations. The elderly were seen as the cornerstone of society in many civilizations, passing on beliefs, traditions, and rituals to the next generation. But as society has become faster and more reliant on technology, seniors' roles have shifted, and many of them now feel underappreciated and left behind.

The way society perceives aging, however, has changed recently, with a greater focus being placed on being healthy and fit well into one's elderly years. Studies have shown that seniors may benefit from regular exercise by preventing chronic ailments like diabetes, heart disease, and osteoporosis, as well as by improving their mental and cognitive abilities.

Notwithstanding these advantages, maintaining an active lifestyle presents special difficulties for many elderly, such as restricted mobility, persistent pain, and restricted access to fitness centers. Senior Strength Training Exercises That Are Easy and Quick Over 60 takes on these issues head-on by offering a variety of workouts that are readily customizable to meet the requirements and abilities of each person.

Anyone hoping to enhance their general well-being, strength, and health in their later years should acquire a copy of Quick and Easy Strength Training Workouts for Seniors Over 60. Seniors who follow the easy, efficient, and enjoyable exercises in this book may benefit from a number of advantages, including better energy and mobility as well as a lower chance of chronic disease and injury.

Why then wait?

Get a copy of Easy and Quick Strength Training Exercises for Seniors Over 60 to get started on the path to a happier, healthier, and stronger future.

The Importance of Strength Training for Seniors

How to Avoid Bone Fractures

Osteoporosis and decreased bone mass make bone fractures and breaks all too prevalent in the elderly. Exercise has been shown to increase bone density, even if osteoporosis might have other causes and may need medical management. Strength training and aerobic weightlifting improve density and lower the chance of breakage.

Muscle Mass is Increased by Strength Training

The typical adult loses 25% of their muscular mass by the age of 70. And the main causes of this are inactivity and disuse. Exercise of any type may stop this loss and increase muscle mass and strength, but resistance training, strength training, and weight lifting work best.

Enhancing Operational Mobility

Improving general function requires strengthening via exercise. Regular strength training may help older persons walk further, become more mobile, and even lessen their need on walkers and canes.

Developing strength also aids in a variety of other useful actions, such as sitting and bathing. Consequently, this eases life and provides access to a wider range of activities.

Improved composition of the body

Women in particular tend to develop more fat as they age and lose muscular mass. It makes individuals more susceptible to long-term ailments. Strength training is a key component of all forms of exercise that contribute to maintaining a healthy body composition.

Seniors Who Strength Train Gain Mental Health Benefits

Mental well-being is as crucial to aging as physical well-being. You run the risk of developing depression, social isolation, loneliness, and other mental health problems as you age. Gaining strength enhances mood and quality of life while improving mobility and function as well as general health.

Safety Tips and Equipment

It is advisable to consult your healthcare professional to ensure that beginning this, or any fitness regimen, is safe for you. It's possible that your physician may recommend changes for your health.

Finding a location where you can comfortably finish the exercises is the next step. Verify that you can walk about and stretch your arms to the fullest without running into any walls or objects. Take out any little area rugs that might trip you up or cause you to slide. For the floor exercises, you may use a yoga mat if you have one.

Finally, always strive to the best of your abilities. It is not necessary to put excessive effort, particularly at the beginning. Although you should anticipate some degree of difficulty and it is natural to feel your body working, you shouldn't experience pain.

Tools

Resistance bands: These are adaptable and provide different intensities of resistance to promote muscle growth and elasticity.

Dumbbells: You may target various muscle areas with a set of light to medium weight dumbbells by using them for a range of exercises.

Stability ball: When doing different workouts, this helps with balance and core strength.

Yoga mat: When stretching and doing floor exercises, a comfy mat is a must.

Foam roller: This is useful for self-massage and for relieving tightness and tension in the muscles.

Ankle weights: You may use them to increase the resistance while doing leg workouts.

Chair or bench: You may use a strong chair or bench as a support for standing workouts or as a place to work when sitting.

Exercise gloves: When utilizing weights or resistance bands, they may aid with grip and reduce the risk of calluses.

Total Time: 25 minutes (5-minute warm-up, 15 minutes strength training, 5-minute cool-down)

Level: Beginner to intermediate

Equipment Needed: Dumbbells or portable weights (3 to 5 pounds to start, 8 to 10 pounds as you grow stronger) are required pieces of equipment. Use common household objects like soup cans or water bottles in place of weights if you don't have any.

What to Expect: When you initially start out, do the exercises without any weight at all if you are a novice. Just concentrate on mastering the movements with proper form. For the exercises that call for it, add dumbbells or another kind of resistance after you are comfortable with each movement.

Warm-Up: 5 Minutes

It is essential to acclimate. Your blood vessels widen while you warm up, which facilitates the flow of oxygen to your muscles. To reduce the strain on your heart, a warm-up also gradually increases heart rate.

Perform each of the next four warm-up exercises for about one minute. Take a few seconds to relax if necessary, but try not to stop in between each movement.

Jog in Place: 1 Minute

For one minute, march while keeping your knees up if low-impact exercise is more comfortable for you.

Punching: 1 Minute

Punching is a fantastic technique to increase blood flow throughout the body and warm up the upper body.

Place your feet slightly more widely than shoulder-width apart and flex your knees a little. To maintain your center of gravity, tighten your core. Punch out at a steady speed, one arm at a time.

Knee Thrusters: 1 Minute

Place your feet wider than shoulder-width apart when starting off, then rotate both of them in the same direction, letting your hips to follow suit as you would in a shallow lunge. The rear heel is elevated and the front knee is at a 90-degree angle. The arms are positioned in front of the chest like a guard.

Raise the rear knee to hip level and press the hands inside against the thigh. Replicate with the foot back on the ground.

Basic Squat: 1 Minute

Do one basic squat to wrap up your warm-up. To maintain the range of motion in your hip flexors, try lowering your glutes as far as you can.

Place your feet hip-distance apart and stand tall. All of your toes, knees, and hips should point forward. As if you were about to recline back onto a chair, bend your knees and stretch your buttocks back. Maintain your weight on your heels and your knees on your toes. Get back up on your feet.

The Workout: 15 Minutes

Perform the suggested number of repetitions for each of the following exercises. Take a minute off after every activity.

Squat Curl Knee Lift

Targets: Biceps, glutes, quads

Beginning in a squat, place your weight back on your heels and extend your arms behind you while gripping dumbbells.
Curl the weights to your shoulders while using your glutes to thrust up and raise your right knee.
After lowering the weights gradually, go back to your squat stance. Continue with your left knee.
Reps: 8–12 on each side

Safety Advice

As you sit into each squat repetition, make an effort to maintain a straight back and an open chest. As you curl, keep the elbows tight to the rib cage.

Shoulder Overhead Press

Targets: Shoulders

Put your feet hip-distance apart to begin. With your arms extended to form a goal post posture, your dumbbells at your sides, and your abs tense, bring your elbows out to the side.
Raise the dumbbells gradually until your arms are straight. Return to your starting location carefully and slowly. For the required amount of repetitions, repeat.
Perform half of the repetitions on one foot while standing, then switch to the other foot to increase the intensity and balance.

Reps range from 8 to 12.

Safety Advice

Raise the weights straight up over your shoulders. To avoid the back arching, try not to let the arms drift back. Try doing this exercise while sitting if you find it difficult to maintain proper posture.

Renegade Arm Row

Targets: shoulders, back, and triceps

Beginning with your legs together, sit back into a small squat while contracting your abs. Dumbbells are held at hip height with the palms facing the ceiling by the arms extended in front of the torso.
Pull elbows back beyond hips, softly embracing the side body, until you feel your triceps and lats contract, then manage the return forward motion.

Reps range from 8 to 12.

Safety Advice

Aim to maintain a neutral spine throughout this movement. Avoid arching the back or bending the spine. A few feet in front of your toes, maintain your attention on the floor.

Bird Dog

Targets: core, glutes, and back

On all fours, kneel on the floor (if you have an exercise mat handy). Extend the other leg behind you, pull in your abdominals, and reach one arm out long.
Continue on the other side.

Reps: 8–10 on each side

Safety Advice

Move steadily and slowly, extending your arm and leg for a little period of time before switching.

Glute Bridge

Targets: Hamstrings and glutes

Lay flat on your back with your feet stacked under your knees and your knees bent hip-distance apart.
As you raise your hips to a bridge, contract your glutes and engage your core. Squeeze tightly and return to the mat in a controlled manner.
Try this exercise with one leg at a time to make it more difficult. Exert the non-working leg while raising and lowering the hips.

Reps range from 8 to 12.

Safety Advice

To protect your neck during this maneuver, keep your eyes focused on the ceiling.

Kneeling Shoulder Tap Push Up

Targets: Arms, shoulders, core

With your back stretched all the way to your knees and your hands on the floor under your shoulders, begin in the kneeling plank position.

Keeping your abs taut, lower your chest to the floor. Tap your right hand on your left shoulder as you lift yourself back up to the kneeling plank, then release it.

Repeat the push-up, but this time, touch your right shoulder with your left hand as you stand up. As you tap, keep your abs firm and resist the urge to tilt your body to one side.

Reps: a total of 8–12 pushups

Safety Advice

For this exercise, if your knees hurt, put a folded blanket below them.

Mid-Back Extension

Targets: Back, core

Place yourself facedown on the mat. To work your abs, lift them off the surface and glide your shoulders down your back. The head raises in a brief hover. You are one continuous line.

As you exhale, pull your chest away from the mat into extension using your core and back muscles. Consider extending from the head's crown.

Breathe in and carefully lower yourself back to the mat, lengthening your spine in the process.

Reps range from 8 to 12.

Safety Advice

If this motion hurts your back, don't do it. You may make the workout more challenging by doing it with your arms extended in front of you like Superman, if your back feels well.

Full Body Sit-Up

Targets: Core, shoulders, back

Begin by reclining on a mat with your feet flexed, your legs stretched, and your arms aloft.
Take a breath, raise your arms, and curve your chin and chest forward. Breathe out while rolling your whole body up and over your legs, maintaining your abs, and reaching your toes.
Breathe in as you start to roll your spine back down, one vertebra at a time, and release as your arms reach above and your upper back lowers. Repeat utilizing your abs to raise and lower yourself rather than your momentum while moving gently.

Reps: eight to ten

Safety Advice

Should you find this uncomfortable on your back, try doing an abdominal crunch while bending your knees. Put your hands behind your head and curl your upper body off the floor while keeping your feet level on the ground. Return to the lower position and repeat.

Cool Down

To lower your heart rate and return to regular breathing, give yourself five minutes. To unwind and complete your exercise, take a few quick walks around the room or in place, or do some basic full-body stretches.

Upper Body Workouts

Wall Push-ups

Target: Shoulders, triceps, and chest

Directions: Place your feet shoulder-width apart and face a wall. With your hands shoulder-width apart and shoulder height above the wall, place them there. Lean your body toward the wall, bending your elbows, and then push yourself back to the starting position.

Reps: 3 sets of ten to fifteen reps

Safety Advice: Maintain a straight line from your head to your heels and a firm core. Keep your hips from protruding or sagging.

Chair Dips

Target: Triceps, Shoulders, and Chest

Instructions: Take a seat with your hands clutching the edge of a solid chair. Step your feet out in front of you, then bend your elbows until they are at a 90-degree angle to lower your body. Return to the starting position by pushing up.

Reps: 3 sets of ten to fifteen reps

Safety Advice: Keep your shoulders back and your ears apart. Keep your elbows from extending out to the sides.

Resistance Band Rows

Target: Biceps and back

Instructions: Hold the grips of a resistance band with your palms facing each other and anchor it at a low position. Pull the handles in the direction of your body and squeeze your shoulder blades together after taking a step back until the band is tight.

Reps: 3 sets of ten to fifteen reps

Safety Advice: Maintain a straight back and a firm core. Avoid hunching over or arching your back.

Dumbbell Curls

Target: Biceps

Directions: Hold a dumbbell in each hand, palms facing front, while standing with your feet shoulder-width apart. Curl the dumbbells in the direction of your shoulders while keeping your upper arms still, then return them to their initial position.

Reps: 3 sets of ten to fifteen reps

Safety Advice: Avoid swinging the weights or lifting them with your momentum. Keep your upper arms still and your elbows tucked in.

Shoulder Press

Target: Triceps and shoulders

Directions: Hold a dumbbell at shoulder height in each hand, palms facing front, while standing with your feet shoulder-width apart. Once your arms are completely extended, press the weights up until they return to their original position.

Reps: 3 sets of ten to fifteen reps

Safety Advice: Avoid bending over or arching your back while pushing the weights. Maintain a rigid core and a straight back.

Arm Circles

Target: Arms and shoulders

Directions: Take a stance with your feet shoulder-width apart, then raise your arms to shoulder height. With your arms, move in little circles, first in one direction and then the other.

Reps: Three sets, ten to fifteen repetitions per direction

Safety Advice: Keep your shoulders down and away from your ears, and keep your arms straight. Avoid swaying your body in order to create circles.

Chest Press

Target: Shoulders, triceps, and chest

Instructions: Place your feet flat on the floor while lying on a bench. Hold a dumbbell at chest height in each hand, with the palms facing front. Once your arms are completely extended, press the weights up until they return to their original position.

Reps: 3 sets of ten to fifteen reps

Safety Advice: Avoid lifting your hips off the bench or hunching your back. Remain flat on your back and your core taut.

Bicep Curls

Target: Biceps

Directions: Hold a dumbbell in each hand, palms facing front, while standing with your feet shoulder-width apart. Curl the dumbbells in the direction of your shoulders while keeping your upper arms still, then return them to their initial position.

Reps: 3 sets of ten to fifteen reps

Safety Advice: Avoid swinging the weights or lifting them with your momentum. Keep your upper arms still and your elbows tucked in.

Tricep Kickbacks

Target: Triceps

Instructions: Hold a dumbbell in each hand with your palms facing your body. Target: Triceps. Maintain a straight back while bending forward at the waist. Return your arms to their maximum length and return the weights to their initial position.

Reps: 3 sets of ten to fifteen reps

Safety Advice: Avoid swinging the weights or hunching over. Maintain a rigid core and a straight back.

Plank

Target: Core

Instructions: Place your elbows just beneath your shoulders as you drop your forearms to the ground from a push-up posture. Maintain a straight posture from your head to your heels and stay there.

Hold for 3 sets of 30–60 seconds for each rep.

Safety Advice: Maintain a firm core and align your hips with your shoulders. Keep your hips from sticking out or sagging.

Lower Body Workouts

Lat Pulldown

Target: The latissimus dorsi, a muscle in the back

Instructions: Place your knees under the pads while seated at the lat pulldown machine. Resuming your starting posture, take a wide grasp on the bar and draw it down to your upper chest.

Reps: 3 sets of ten to fifteen reps

Safety Advice: Throughout the workout, avoid arching your back and maintain a straight back. Avoid using excessive weight that might put pressure on your back or shoulders.

Seated Cable Row

Target: Back muscles, including the latissimus dorsi and rhomboids

Directions: Take a seat at the cable row machine, place your feet on the footrests, and use an overhand hold on the handle. Return to the beginning position after pulling the handle in the direction of your abdomen.

Reps: 3 sets of ten to fifteen reps

Safety Advice: Throughout the exercise, maintain a straight back and refrain from curving it. Avoid using excessive weight that might put pressure on your back or shoulders.

Chest Fly

Target: Chest muscles, specifically the pectoralis major

Directions: Hold a dumbbell in each hand while lying flat on a bench. With your palms facing each other, raise your arms straight up. Return to the beginning posture after lowering the dumbbells out to the sides while bending your elbows just a little.

Reps: 3 sets of ten to fifteen reps

Safety Advice: Avoid using excessive weight that can put pressure on your chest or shoulders. Throughout the exercise, keep your elbows slightly bent to prevent hyperextension.

Incline Dumbbell Press

Target: Chest muscles, specifically the upper portion of the pectoralis major

Directions: Hold a dumbbell in each hand while seated on an inclined bench. Maintaining a small bend in your elbows, press the dumbbells up over your chest and then drop them to the sides of your chest.

Reps: 3 sets of ten to fifteen reps

Safety Advice: Avoid using excessive weight that can put pressure on your chest or shoulders. Throughout the exercise, keep your back flat on the bench and refrain from arching it.

Reverse Fly

Target: Back muscles, specifically the rear deltoids and rhomboids

Directions: Bend forward at the waist while maintaining a straight back. Stand with your feet shoulder-width apart. With your hands facing each other, hold a dumbbell in each hand. Stretch your arms out to the sides and then take a step back to the beginning.

Reps: 3 sets of ten to fifteen reps

Safety Advice: Avoid using excessive weight that can put stress on your back or shoulders. Throughout the exercise, keep your back straight and refrain from curving it.

Lateral Raise

Target: The lateral deltoids, which are shoulder muscles

Directions: Hold a dumbbell in each hand with the palms facing your body while standing with your feet shoulder-width apart. Return to the beginning posture after raising your arms out to the sides until they are parallel to the floor.

Reps: 3 sets of ten to fifteen reps

Safety Advice: Avoid using excessive weight that can put pressure on your shoulders. Throughout the exercise, keep your back straight and refrain from arching it.

Hammer Curls

Target: Biceps

Directions: Hold a dumbbell in each hand with the palms facing your body while standing with your feet shoulder-width apart. Curl the dumbbells up to your shoulders while keeping your elbows close to your sides, then take a step back to the beginning position.

Reps: 3 sets of ten to fifteen reps

Safety Advice: Avoid using excessive weight that might put stress on your shoulders or arms. Throughout the workout, maintain a straight back and refrain from flailing your arms.

Tricep Pushdown

Target: Triceps

Directions: Face the cable machine with the straight bar attachment facing you. With an overhand grip, stretch your arms completely by pushing down on the bar, then take a step back to the starting position.

Reps: 3 sets of ten to fifteen reps

Safety Advice: Avoid using excessive weight that might put stress on your shoulders or arms. Throughout the exercise, keep your back straight and refrain from arching it.

Overhead Tricep Extension

Target: Triceps

Directions: Hold a dumbbell over your head with both hands while standing with your feet shoulder-width apart. Return to the beginning posture after lowering the weight behind your head while maintaining your elbows near to your ears.

Reps: 3 sets of ten to fifteen reps

Safety Advice: Avoid using excessive weight that might put stress on your shoulders or arms. Throughout the exercise, keep your back straight and refrain from arching it.

Face Pull

Target: Back muscles, specifically the rear deltoids and rhomboids

Steps to follow: Face a cable machine that has a rope attachment. Using an overhand hold, grab the rope and pull it in the direction of your face. Then, go back to the beginning position.

Reps: 3 sets of ten to fifteen reps

Safety Advice: Avoid using excessive weight that might put stress on your shoulders or arms. Throughout the exercise, keep your back straight and refrain from arching it.

Core and Balance Exercises

Bird Dog

Target: Core, back, and glutes

Directions: Extend your left arm and right leg at the same time, starting on your hands and knees. After a brief period of holding, go back to the initial position. Continue on the other side.

Repetitions: 10 repetitions on each side, in three sets.

Safety Advice: Maintain a straight back and a firm core. Avoid sagging your hips or hunching your back.

Single-Leg Stand

Target: Balance and leg strength

Directions: Take a single leg stand and maintain it for as long as you can. Repeat after switching legs.
3 sets of 30–60 seconds for each leg of the reps

Safety Advice: If you need assistance, use a chair or wall. Maintain a rigid core and a straight back. Avert locking of the knee.

Side Leg Raises

Target: Hips and outer thighs

Directions: Stack your legs while lying on your right side. Raise and then return your left leg to its starting position. Continue on the other side.

Repetitions: 10 repetitions on each side, in three sets.

Safety Advice: Avoid twisting or hunching your back. Maintain a tight core and stacked hips.

Seated Leg Lifts

Target: Core and hip flexors

Directions: Take a seat and place your feet flat on the floor. Raise one leg, then bring it back down. Continue on the other side.

Repetitions: 10 repetitions on each side, in three sets.

Safety Advice: Avoid hunching over or arching your back. Maintain a rigid core and a straight back.

Standing Marches

Target: Core, balance, and leg strength

Steps to follow: Place your feet shoulder-width apart. Raise one knee to your chest and then return it to its original position. Continue on the other side.

Repetitions: 10 repetitions on each side, in three sets.

Safety Advice: Maintain a straight back and a firm core. Avoid hunching over or arching your back.

Heel-to-Toe Walk

Target: Balance and leg strength

Directions: Step forward, heel to toe, putting one foot in front of the other. Step forward, keeping a straight line of sight between your feet.

Repetitions: 10 repetitions on each side, in three sets.

Safety Advice: If you require assistance, use a chair or wall. Maintain a rigid core and a straight back. Avert locking of the knee.

Standing Hip Extensions

Target: Glutes and lower back

Steps to follow: Place your feet shoulder-width apart. Raise a leg and then bring it back down. Continue on the other side.

Repetitions: 10 repetitions on each side, in three sets.

Safety Advice: Maintain a straight back and a firm core. Avoid hunching over or bending forward.

Seated Leg Circles

Target: Core and hip flexors

Directions: Take a seat and place your feet flat on the floor. Raise one leg and use your foot to create little circles. Continue on the other side.

Repetitions: 10 repetitions on each side, in three sets.

Safety Advice: Avoid hunching over or arching your back. Maintain a rigid core and a straight back.

Standing Knee Lifts

Target: Core and balance

Steps to follow: Place your feet shoulder-width apart. Raise one knee to your chest and then return it to its original position. Continue on the other side.

Repetitions: 10 repetitions on each side, in three sets.

Safety Advice: Maintain a straight back and a firm core. Avoid hunching over or arching your back.

Modified V-Sits

Target: Core

Directions: Take a seat on the ground with your feet flat on the floor and your knees bent. Raise your feet off the floor and slant your back a little. Keep the job.

Reps: three 30- to 60-second sets

Safety Advice: Avoid hunching over or straining your neck. Maintain a rigid core and a straight back.

Please wait, Your Review is Very Important…

Dear Reader,

I hope this message finds you well. Thank you for choosing to read the **Quick and Simple Strength Training Workouts for Seniors Over 60**. Your feedback is incredibly valuable to me, and I would love to hear your thoughts on the book. Whether you've just started, are halfway through, or have finished reading, your perspective matters.

Your feedback is immensely appreciated and will help me enhance future works.

Thank you for taking the time to share your thoughts on **Quick and Simple Strength Training Workouts for Seniors Over 60**. Your support means the world to me.

Happy reading!

Carol Bolden

Flexibility and Posture Exercises

Shoulder Rolls

Target: Upper back and shoulders

Directions: Take a seat or stand with your arms casually by your sides. Make a complete circle with your shoulders by gently rolling them forward. Proceed in the other direction and repeat the action.

Reps: 10 to 15 in each way

Safety Advice: Avoid shrugging your shoulders up to your ears and move slowly and deliberately.

Neck Stretches

Target: Neck muscles and upper back

Directions: Tilt your head slightly to the side and place your ear on your shoulder. After holding for 15 to 30 seconds, switch to the other side.

Reps: two to three times per side

Safety advice: Move slowly and deliberately; steer clear of jerky or abrupt motions.

Chest Expansion

Target: Chest and shoulder muscles

Instructions: Squeeze your shoulder blades together, raise your arms gently, and clasp your hands behind your back. Release after holding for 15 to 30 seconds.

Reps: two to three

Safety Advice: Avoid straining your neck or arching your back by maintaining a straight back and an engaged core.

Hip Flexor Stretch

Target: Hip flexors and quads

Instructions: Put your other foot flat on the ground in front of you and kneel on one knee. Till the front of your rear leg stretches, gently drive your hips forward. After holding for 15 to 30 seconds, swap sides.

Reps: two to three times per side

Safety Advice: Avoid bending forward or arching your back; instead, maintain a straight back and an engaged core.

Hamstring Stretch

Target: Hamstrings and lower back

Directions: Take a seat on a chair and put one leg out in front of you. Maintain a straight back as you extend your hand toward your toes. After holding for 15 to 30 seconds, swap your legs.

Reps: two to three times per leg

Safety Advice: Avoid jumping or jerking your leg, and maintain a straight back and engaged core.

Calf Stretch

Target: Calves and ankles

Directions: Put one leg behind you while facing a wall. Lean forward while maintaining your rear leg straight and your heel planted on the ground. After holding for 15 to 30 seconds, swap your legs.

Reps: two to three times per leg

Safety advice: Don't lock your knee or overextend your foot, and maintain a straight back and a strong core.

Spinal Twist

Target: Lower back and core muscles

Directions: Take a seat and place your feet flat on the floor. Using the chair's arm to extend the stretch, slowly rotate your body to one side. After holding for 15 to 30 seconds, swap sides.

Reps: two to three times per side

Safety Advice: Avoid twisting too sharply or too rapidly, and maintain a straight back and engaged core.

Seated Leg Extensions

Target: Quads and hip flexors

Directions: Take a seat and place your feet flat on the floor. Raise one leg off the floor while maintaining a straight knee. After holding for 15 to 30 seconds, swap your legs.

Reps: two to three times per leg

Safety Advice: Avoid bending forward or arching your back; instead, maintain a straight back and an engaged core.

Arm Circles

Target: Shoulders and upper back

Directions: Arrange your feet so that they are shoulder-width apart, then spread your arms out to the sides. Using your arms, make little circles that progressively become bigger.

Reps: 10 to 15 in each way

Safety Advice: Avoid straining your neck or arching your back by maintaining a straight back and an engaged core.

Cat-Cow

Target: Lower back and core muscles

Directions: Lie flat on your back and begin on your hands and knees. Lower your belly to the ground (like a cow) and gently arch your back upward (like a cat). For 15 to 30 seconds, repeat this procedure.

Reps: ten to fifteen times

Safety Advice: Avoid putting too much pressure on your neck or back by keeping your back straight and your core active.

Sample Workout Plans

Are you prepared to start a 30-day adventure that will lead to a more active and healthful lifestyle? The goal of this exercise program is to enhance functional strength, mobility, and general well-being in seniors and older people. A variety of exercises are included in the program to target different muscle groups and to help with endurance, flexibility, and balance.

Remember to speak with your healthcare provider before beginning to be sure the workouts are suitable for your particular requirements and capabilities.

Week 1: Getting Started

Make sure you get into a pattern and get comfortable with the workouts throughout the first week. Every exercise should start with a 5-minute warm-up, which may be something as simple as a light arm circular or a march in place.

Day 1:

- Shoulder Rolls: 10 reps
- Neck Stretches: 3 reps on each side
- Chest Expansion: 3 reps
- Hip Flexor Stretch: 3 reps on each side
- Hamstring Stretch: 3 reps on each side
- Calf Stretch: 3 reps on each side
- Spinal Twist: 3 reps on each side

- Seated Leg Extensions: 10 reps on each side
- Arm Circles: 10 reps in each direction
- Cat-Cow: 10 reps

Day 2: Rest

Day 3: Repeat Day 1

Day 4: Rest

Day 5: Repeat Day 1

Day 6: Rest

Day 7: Rest

Week 2: Building Strength

In the second week, carry over the activities from the first week and include the following strength-training exercises:

Day 8:

- Wall Push-ups: 10 reps
- Chair Dips: 10 reps
- Resistance Band Rows: 10 reps
- Dumbbell Curls: 10 reps
- Shoulder Press: 10 reps
- Arm Circles: 10 reps in each direction
- Chest Press: 10 reps

- Bicep Curls: 10 reps
- Tricep Kickbacks: 10 reps
- Plank: 30 seconds

Day 9: Rest

Day 10: Repeat Day 8

Day 11: Rest

Day 12: Repeat Day 8

Day 13: Rest

Day 14: Rest

Week 3: Increasing Endurance

In the third week, carry over the workouts from the first two weeks and include the following endurance-enhancing activities:

Day 15:

- Bird Dog: 10 reps on each side
- Single-Leg Stand: 3 reps on each side
- Side Leg Raises: 10 reps on each side
- Seated Leg Lifts: 10 reps on each side
- Standing Marches: 30 seconds
- Heel-to-Toe Walk: 30 seconds

- Standing Hip Extensions: 10 reps
- Seated Leg Circles: 10 reps on each side
- Standing Knee Lifts: 10 reps on each side
- Modified V-Sits: 30 seconds

Day 16: Rest

Day 17: Repeat Day 15

Day 18: Rest

Day 19: Repeat Day 15

Day 20: Rest

Day 21: Rest

Week 4: Enhancing Balance and Flexibility

Incorporate the following balance and flexibility exercises into the workouts from Weeks 1-3 during the fourth and final week:

Day 22:

- Wall Push-ups: 10 reps
- Chair Dips: 10 reps
- Resistance Band Rows: 10 reps
- Dumbbell Curls: 10 reps
- Shoulder Press: 10 reps
- Arm Circles: 10 reps in each direction

- Chest Press: 10 reps
- Bicep Curls: 10 reps
- Tricep Kickbacks: 10 reps
- Plank: 30 seconds
- Bird Dog: 10 reps on each side
- Single-Leg Stand: 3 reps on each side
- Side Leg Raises: 10 reps on each side
- Seated Leg Lifts: 10 reps on each side
- Standing Marches: 30 seconds
- Heel-to-Toe Walk: 30 seconds
- Standing Hip Extensions: 10 reps
- Seated Leg Circles: 10 reps on each side
- Standing Knee Lifts: 10 reps on each side
- Modified V-Sits: 30 seconds

Day 23: Rest

Day 24: Repeat Day 22

Day 25: Rest

Day 26: Repeat Day 22

Day 27: Rest

Day 28: Rest

Week 5: The Final Stretch

In the last week, go on with the exercises from Weeks 1-4 and push yourself farther by adding these exercises:

Day 29:

- Wall Push-ups: 15 reps
- Chair Dips: 15 reps
- Resistance Band Rows: 15 reps
- Dumbbell Curls: 15 reps
- Shoulder Press: 15 reps
- Arm Circles: 15 reps in each direction
- Chest Press: 15 reps
- Bicep Curls: 15 reps
- Tricep Kickbacks: 15 reps
- Plank: 45 seconds
- Bird Dog: 15 reps on each side
- Single-Leg Stand: 4 reps on each side
- Side Leg Raises: 15 reps on each side
- Seated Leg Lifts: 15 reps on each side
- Standing Marches: 45 seconds
- Heel-to-Toe Walk: 45 seconds
- Standing Hip Extensions: 15 reps
- Seated Leg Circles: 15 reps on each side
- Standing Knee Lifts: 15 reps on each side
- Modified V-Sits: 45 seconds

Day 30: Rest

Best wishes! Congratulations! You've finished the 30-Day Active Aging Fitness Program. Remind yourself to keep up your normal exercise schedule and to speak with a healthcare provider if you have any questions or concerns about it.

Progress Tracking and Goal Setting

Maintain a diary for your workouts: Jot down the movements, repetitions, sets, and weights you employ in each workout. This will enable you to track your development and modify your exercise regimen as necessary.

Establish SMART objectives: Ensure that your objectives are Specific, Measurable, Achievable, Relevant, and Time-bound. Say "I want to get stronger," for instance, but instead make a goal like "I want to increase my bench press by 10 pounds in 3 months."

Utilize an app for fitness: You may create objectives, keep track of your exercises, and assess your progress using a variety of applications. Popular choices include of JEFIT, Fitbod, and Strong.

Speak with an expert: See a personal trainer or physical therapist if you're unclear about how to measure your progress or establish reasonable objectives. They are able to provide helpful advice and assistance.

Remain patient: Keep in mind that development takes time, particularly as we age. Have patience with yourself and acknowledge your little accomplishments as you go.

Nutrition and Lifestyle Tips

The secret to maximizing the benefits of strength training is a well-balanced diet. To help you maximize the benefits of your exercise, consider the following dietary advice:

Make protein a priority. To assist muscle development and repair, aim for 1.2 to 2.0 grams of protein per kilogram of body weight each day.

To avoid dehydration and preserve peak performance, stay hydrated by drinking plenty of water before to, during, and after your exercises.

Select complete foods: To promote general health, choose nutrient-dense, whole foods including fruits, vegetables, whole grains, lean protein, and healthy fats.

Consume enough calories. Make sure you're eating enough calories to maintain your current level of exercise and avoid losing muscle.

Speak with a certified dietitian: If you need assistance creating a customized eating plan, you may want to engage with a registered dietitian with experience in senior nutrition.

Lifestyle Suggestions

A balanced diet and well-rounded workout regimen are important, but there are other lifestyle choices that may help your strength training efforts succeed as well:

Get adequate sleep: To promote general health and muscular recovery, aim for 7-9 hours of good sleep per night.

Control your stress: Take up stress-relieving exercises like yoga, deep breathing, or meditation to assist manage your stress levels.

Remain socially connected: To keep motivated and socially engaged, make sure you have close relationships with your friends and family. You may also want to join a club or class that focuses on strength training.

Maintain coherence: As much as possible, follow your diet and exercise plan, and keep in mind that long-term success depends on consistency.

How to Overcome Common Challenges

Make sure your objectives are concise, attainable, and grounded in reality. Divide them into more achievable, smaller goals to help you stay motivated and focused.

Maintain coherence: When it comes to reaching your fitness objectives, consistency is essential. Maintain and turn your exercise regimen into a habit. Recall that results take time to manifest, so exercise patience and persevere!

Warm up and cool down: You may avoid injuries and enhance your performance by warming up before an exercise session and cooling down afterwards. Make sure your warm-up consists of dynamic stretches and mild cardio, and your cool-down consists of static stretches.

Pay attention to your body. During your exercises, pay attention to any aches or pains you may feel. If anything doesn't feel quite right, halt and get expert advice. Being safe is preferable to being sorry!

Change things up: Use a variety of exercises and activities to keep your training engaging. You'll be more motivated and avoid boredom if you do this.

Drink plenty of water and eat a healthy diet. These are prerequisites for both peak performance and recuperation. A balanced diet full of healthy foods and plenty of water should be followed.

Give your body the time it needs to relax and heal so that it can restore itself. Aside from getting enough sleep, remember to include rest days in your exercise regimen.

Remain upbeat and enjoy yourself: Recall to relish the journey and acknowledge and appreciate your accomplishments, no matter how little. Maintaining focus and conquering obstacles may be greatly aided by having a good attitude and a sense of humor.

Please wait, Your Review is Very Important…

Dear Reader,

I hope this message finds you well. Thank you for choosing to read the **Quick and Simple Strength Training Workouts for Seniors Over 60**. Your feedback is incredibly valuable to me, and I would love to hear your thoughts on the book. Whether you've just started, are halfway through, or have finished reading, your perspective matters.

Your feedback is immensely appreciated and will help me enhance future works.

Thank you for taking the time to share your thoughts on **Quick and Simple Strength Training Workouts for Seniors Over 60**. Your support means the world to me.

Happy reading!

Carol Bolden

Conclusion

By the time this insightful trip comes to a close, we hope you have realized just how amazing strength training is for seniors over 60. You are making a big improvement to your general health and well-being by adding these short and easy exercises into your daily regimen.

We have discussed the significance of preserving posture, strength, and flexibility as we age throughout this book. These 20 minutes of intense training have improved your physical skills while also increasing your self-assurance and independence.

Never forget that you may always begin your fitness journey at any time. You have shown resiliency, tenacity, and a dedication to a better future with every exercise. You'll discover that the outcomes speak for themselves if you stick with these activities.

You have the ability to rewrite the definition of what it means to age gracefully as a senior. You are demonstrating that age is nothing more than a number and pushing the boundaries of aging with each stride, stretch, and lift. Accept your increased strength and flexibility and keep motivating others to start their own fitness adventures.

Finally, we would want to thank you for coming along on this journey with us. We hope that this book has given you the information and resources you need to improve your health and wellbeing in the long run. As you continue to work so hard toward your fitness objectives, never forget that the possibilities are endless!

YOUR VIDEO COURSE IS RIGHT HERE!!!

Kindly type in the link in your browser to gain access, thank you.

A Full Course Playlist:

http://tinyurl.com/3wae6xaf

OR

Scan the QR code below: